21-DAY DIETING FOR OBESITY

Transform Your Health with Simple, Effective, and Sustainable Plan

BY AURORA GRACE

DEDICATION

To all who are struggling with obesity and seeking a healthier life,

This book is dedicated to you brave individuals ready to take control of your health and well being. As you embark on this 21-day journey, remember that each step brings you closer to:

1. Reducing risk of heart disease and stroke
2. Low blood pressure and cholesterol levels
3. Improving mobility and less joint pain
4. Good sleep quality and increased energy
5. Enhanced self-esteem and mental well-being

May this book guide you towards sustainable weight loss and a vibrant, healthy life. Your courage to change inspires us.

With heartfelt appreciation to all professionals,
nutritionists, and successful weight loss achievers who
shared their expertise and experiences.

Your transformation starts now.

TABLE OF CONTENTS

1.INTRODUCTION Understanding Obesity

2. WEEK1: Kickstarting Your Journey

3. WEEK 2: Building Healthy Habits

4. WEEK3: Achieving and Sustaining Results

5. Exercise and Physical Activity

6. Mindset and Motivation

7. Real-Life Success Stories

8. Additional Resources

9. Conclusion

Celebrating Your Progress

10. Measurement Conversion Charts

THANK YOU!

Bonus

11.7-Day Healthy Habit Booster Plan

INTRODUCTION

Transforming your health with Simple, Effective and Sustainable Plan.This book is designed to provide you with a comprehensive and easy-to-follow plan that will help take control of your weight, improve your health, and transform your life. Let's embark on this journey together, starting with an understanding of obesity and the importance of a structured diet plan.

Understanding Obesity: Causes and Consequences

Obesity is a complex and multifaceted health condition that affects millions of people worldwide. It occurs when excess body fat accumulates to the extent that it may have a negative impact on health. The causes of obesity are diverse and can include:

Genetics: Your genes can affect how your body processes food and stores fat.
Lifestyle: Poor eating habits, lack of physical activity, and sedentary behaviours contribute significantly to weight gain.

Environment: Access to unhealthy foods, lack of safe areas for exercise, and other environmental factors can influence your weight.

Factors: Stress, emotional eating, and certain mental health conditions can lead to overeating and weight gain.

Medical Conditions: Some medical issues and medications can cause weight gain or make it harder to lose weight.

The consequences of obesity are serious and can include an increased risk of developing chronic diseases such as type 2 diabetes, heart disease, stroke, and certain types of cancer. Additionally, obesity can impact mental health, leading to conditions such as depression and anxiety. Understanding these causes and consequences is the first step toward making meaningful changes to your lifestyle and health.

The Importance of a Structured Diet Plan

A structured diet plan is essential for managing obesity and achieving lasting weight loss. Here's why:

Accountability: A structured plan helps you stay accountable to your goals, making it easier to track your progress and stay motivated.

Balanced Nutrition: It ensures that you receive a balanced intake of essential nutrients, avoiding the pitfalls of fad diets that can lead to nutritional deficiencies.

Portion Control: Learning to control portion sizes is crucial for managing calorie intake and preventing overeating.

Sustainable Habits: A well-designed plan promotes the development of healthy, sustainable eating habits that can be maintained long-term, rather than temporary fixes.

Personalization: A good plan can be tailored to fit your individual needs, preferences, and lifestyle, making it easier to stick with.

How This 21-Day Plan Will Help An Obese person.

Our 21-day dieting plan is specifically crafted to help you lose weight in a healthy and sustainable way.

Step-by-Step Guidance: Each day of the plan is outlined with clear instructions, meal plans, and recipes, making it easy to follow.

Educational Content: Learn about the importance of nutrition, how to make healthier food choices, and the impact of different foods on your body.

Holistic Approach: The plan includes not just diet but also tips for physical activity, mindset, and motivation, addressing all aspects of weight management.

Flexibility: While the plan is structured, it allows for flexibility and personalization to suit your individual needs and preferences.

Long-Term Success: By the end of the 21 days, you'll have developed new habits and a better understanding of how to maintain your weight loss and continue on your journey to better health.

WEEK 1

Kickstarting Your Journey

DAY 1-3: Understanding Your Body and Setting Goals

The initial stage of the 21-day journey is all about understanding your body, recognizing your unique needs, and setting realistic, achievable goals.

DAY 1: Understanding Your Body

Self-Assessment: Take time to assess your current eating habits, lifestyle, and physical activity. Understanding where you are starting from will help you set realistic goals.

Measurements: Record your starting weight, measurements, and take a photo. This will help you track your progress and stay motivated.

Mindset: Reflect on your relationship with food and identify any emotional triggers that lead to overeating. A positive mindset is crucial for success.

DAY 2: Setting Realistic Goals

Goal Setting: Set SMART (Specific, Measurable, Achievable, Relevant, Time-bound) goals for the next 21 days. For example, aim to lose 5 pounds, increase daily physical activity, or eat more vegetables.

Action Plan: Break down your goals into smaller, manageable steps. Write down what you need to do each day to achieve these goals.

DAY 3: Preparing for Success

Meal Planning: Plan your meals for the week ahead. Include a variety of healthy, nutrient-dense foods to keep your diet balanced.

Grocery Shopping: Make a shopping list of the ingredients you'll need and stock up on healthy options.

Support System: Inform friends or family about your goals and ask for their support. Having a support system can greatly increase your chances of success.

DAY 4-7: Eating Clean Basics and Detoxification

Clean eating is about choosing whole, minimally processed foods that nourish your body and support your health. These next few days will help you transition into clean eating habits and start the detoxification process.

DAY 4: Introducing Clean Eating

Whole Foods: Focus on eating whole foods such as fruits, vegetables, lean proteins, whole grains, and healthy fats. Avoid processed foods, sugary snacks, and beverages.

Hydration: Drink plenty of water throughout the day to help your body flush out toxins.

DAY 5: Meal Preparation

Batch Cooking: Prepare and cook meals in batches to save time and ensure you have healthy options available throughout the week.

Healthy Snacks: Keep healthy snacks like cut-up vegetables, fruits, and nuts readily available to avoid reaching for unhealthy options.

DAY 6: Detoxification

Detox Drinks: Incorporate detoxifying drinks such as lemon water, green tea, and smoothies into your daily routine.

Physical Activity: Engage in light physical activity like walking or yoga to support the detox process.

DAY 7: Reflect and Adjust

Evaluate: Reflect on your progress and how you're feeling. Adjust your meal plans and goals as needed.

Celebrate: Celebrate your small victories and stay motivated for the weeks ahead.

Sample Meal Plans and Recipes

Breakfast: Green Smoothie

INGREDIENT:
Spinach,
 banana,

almond milk,
chia seed berries.

PREPARATION

1.Blend spinach, banana, and almond milk until smooth.

2.Pour into a bowl and top with chia seeds and berries.

Lunch: Quinoa Salad

INGREDIENTS:
Cooked quinoa
cherry tomatoes
cucumber
chickpeas
feta cheese
olive oil
lemon juice
salt, and pepper

PREPARATION

Combine all ingredients in a bowl and toss with olive oil
and lemon juice. Season with salt and pepper to taste.

Dinner: Grilled Chicken with Vegetables

INGREDIENTS:
Chicken breast,
mixed vegetables (bell peppers, zucchini, broccoli),
olive oil,
garlic,
 herbs.

PREPARATION

 Marinate chicken with olive oil, garlic, and herbs.
 Grill the chicken and vegetables until cooked and served.

Snack: Apple Slices with Almond Butter

INGREDIENTS:
Apple,
almond butter.

PREPARATION

Slice the apple and spread almond butter on each slice for a satisfying and healthy snack serve and enjoy.

Embrace these first seven days with enthusiasm and commitment. You're laying the foundation for a healthier lifestyle and setting yourself up for long-term success. Remember, each step you take brings you closer to your goals. get started.

WEEK 2

Building Healthy Habits

Welcome to Week 2 of your 21-day journey! You've laid a strong foundation in Week 1 by understanding your body and kick starting clean eating habits. Now, it's time to build on that momentum by incorporating balanced nutrition and mastering meal prep and planning. These steps will help you create sustainable, healthy habits that will support your weight loss and overall well-being.

DAY 8-10: Incorporating Balanced Nutrition

Balanced nutrition is crucial for maintaining energy levels, supporting metabolic functions, and achieving your weight loss goals. During these days, we'll focus on creating well-rounded meals that include all the essential nutrients our body needs.

DAY 8: Understanding Macronutrients

Proteins: Essential for muscle repair and growth. Include lean sources like chicken, fish, tofu, and legumes in your meals.

Carbohydrates: Your body's primary energy source. Complex carbs such as whole grains, fruits, and vegetables are to be focused on.

Fats: Necessary for nutrient absorption and hormone production. Always Opt for healthy fats like avocados, nuts, seeds, and olive oil.

DAY 9: Creating Balanced Meals

Proportions: Aim to fill half your plate with vegetables, a quarter with lean protein, and a quarter with whole grains or starchy vegetables.

Variety: Incorporate a variety of foods to ensure you get a range of vitamins and minerals.

Hydration: Continue to drink plenty of water and consider adding herbal teas to your routine for variety

DAY 10: Nutrient Timing

Meal Timing: Eat regular meals and snacks to keep your metabolism steady to prevent overeating.

Pre- and Post-Workout Nutrition: Fuel your workouts with a mix of carbs and proteins, and replenish your energy with a balanced snack afterward.

DAY 11-14: Meal Prep and Planning

Effective meal prep and planning are key to staying on track with your diet. By dedicating time to plan and prepare your meals, you'll save time, reduce stress, and avoid unhealthy food choices.

DAY 11: Planning Your Meals

Weekly Plan: Create a meal plan for the week that includes breakfast, lunch, dinner, and snacks. Make sure it aligns with your nutritional goals.

Shopping List: Always write down all the ingredients needed and stick to your list to avoid impulse buys.

DAY 12: Batch Cooking

Cook in Bulk: Prepare large quantities of staples like grains, proteins, and roasted vegetables. Store them in the fridge or freezer for easy access throughout the week.

Portion Control: Use containers to portion out meals and snacks, making it easier to manage serving sizes.

DAY 13: Quick and Easy Recipes

Simple Meals: Focus on recipes that are quick to prepare but still nutritious. Think stir-fries, salads, and sheet pan dinners.

Healthy Snacks: Prepare snacks like yoghourt with berries, veggie sticks with hummus and homemade trail mix.

DAY 14: Review and Adjust

Evaluate: Look back at your week and assess what worked well and what didn't. Adjust your meal plans and prep strategies as needed.

Stay Flexible: Be open to trying new recipes and ingredients to keep your meals exciting and satisfying.

Sample Meal Plans and Recipes

Breakfast: Overnight Oats

INGREDIENTS:
Rolled oats
 chia seeds
almond milk
honey
fresh berries

PREPARATION

 Mix oats, chia seeds, and almond milk in a jar.
Refrigerate overnight. Add honey and berries before
serving.

Lunch:Mediterranean Quinoa Bowl

INGREDIENTS:
Cooked quinoa,
 cherry tomatoes,
cucumber,
olives,
 feta cheese,
chickpeas,
olive oil,
lemon juice.

PREPARATION

Mix all ingredients in a bowl. Drizzle with olive oil and lemon juice.

Dinner: Baked Salmon with Asparagus

INGREDIENTS:
Salmon fillets,
asparagus,
olive oil,
garlic,
lemon,
 salt,
pepper.

PREPARATION

Preheat the oven to 400°F. Place salmon and asparagus on a baking sheet.
Drizzle with olive oil, and sprinkle with garlic, salt, and pepper.
Bake for 20 minutes. Serve with a squeeze of lemon.

Snack: Greek Yoghourt with Nuts and Honey

INGREDIENTS:
Greek yoghourt,

mixed nuts,
honey.

PREPARATION

Serve Greek yoghourt topped with honey and a mixture
of nuts.

Embrace Week 2 with incorporating balanced nutrition
and mastering meal prep, you're setting yourself up for
long-term success and a healthier lifestyle. Embrace
week 2 Keep going.

WEEK 3

Achieving and Sustaining Results

You have established healthy habits and a solid foundation. Now is the time to concentrate on controlling cravings, overcoming emotional eating, remaining active, and remaining motivated. This week is all about establishing those routines and ensuring success in the long run. This is the last week of your 21-day journey of Dieting.

DAY 15-17: Managing Cravings and Emotional Eating

These next few days will help you develop strategies to manage the challenges effectively. Because cravings

and emotional eating can be major obstacles to
maintaining a healthy weight loss diet.

DAY 15: Understanding Cravings

Identifying Triggers: Pay attention to what triggers your
cravings. Is it stress, boredom, or certain social
situations?

Healthy Alternatives: Find healthier alternatives to your
usual cravings. For example, if you crave something
sweet, opt for fruit or a small piece of dark chocolate.

DAY 16: Emotional Eating

Mindful Eating: Practise mindful eating by paying full
attention to your meals. Eat slowly, savour each bite,
and listen to your body's hunger and fullness cues.

Stress Management: Incorporate stress management
techniques such as meditation, deep breathing, or yoga
to help control emotional eating.

DAY 17: Building a Support System

Seeking Support: Surround yourself with supportive
friends, family, or a community that understands your
goals. Sharing your journey can provide motivation and
accountability.

Professional Help: If emotional eating is a significant issue, consider seeking help from a therapist or a support group.

DAY 18-21: Staying Active and Motivated

Staying active and maintaining motivation are crucial for sustaining your results. These final days focus on integrating physical activity into your routine and keeping your motivation high.

DAY 18: Importance of Physical Activity

Daily Movement: Aim to incorporate some form of physical activity into your daily routine, whether it's a brisk walk, a workout, or a yoga session.

Enjoyable Exercises: Find exercises you enjoy so that staying active feels less like a chore and more like a fun part of your day.

DAY 19: Fitness Setting Goals

Realistic Goals: Set realistic fitness goals that align with your overall health objectives. This could be increasing your daily steps, improving your strength, or enhancing your flexibility.

Track Progress: Use a journal or an app to track your progress and celebrate your achievements, no matter how small.

DAY 20: Staying Motivated

Find Inspiration: Keep yourself motivated by finding inspiration in books, podcasts, or success stories of others who have achieved their health goals.

Reward Yourself: Set up a reward system for reaching milestones. This could be a relaxing spa day, a new workout outfit, or any non-food reward that makes you happy.

DAY 21: Planning and ReflectionAhead

Reflect: Take time to reflect on your journey over the past three weeks. What worked well? What challenges did you overcome?

Plan for the Future: Use what you've learned to plan for the future. Continue setting goals, staying active, and eating mindfully to maintain your progress.

Sample Meal Plans and Recipes

Breakfast: Veggie Omelette

INGREDIENTS:
Eggs,
spinach,
tomatoes,
bell peppers,
onions,
cheese (optional).

PREPARATION

Whisk eggs and pour into a heated pan. Chop vegetables and add, then cook until the eggs are set. Sprinkle with cheese if desired.

Lunch: Chicken and Avocado Salad

INGREDIENTS:
Grilled chicken breast,
mixed greens,
avocado,
cherry tomatoes,
cucumber,
olive oil,
lemon juice.

PREPARATION

Combine all ingredients in a bowl. Drizzle with olive oil and lemon juice. Toss to coat.

Dinner: Stir-Fried Tofu with Vegetables

INGREDIENTS:
 Firm tofu,
broccoli,
bell peppers,
carrots,
soy sauce,
garlic,
ginger,
olive oil.

PREPARATION

Sauté garlic and ginger in olive oil. Add tofu and cook until golden brown. Add vegetables and soy sauce, stir-frying until vegetables are tender.

Snack: Hummus and Veggie Sticks

INGREDIENTS
Carrot sticks,
cucumber sticks,
bell pepper slices,
hummus.

PREPARATION

 Dip the vegetable sticks into hummus for a satisfying and healthy snack.

By managing cravings, staying active, and keeping yourself motivated, you can achieve and sustain your weight loss and health improvements in your 21-day journey.

EXERCISE AND PHYSICAL ACTIVITY

Physical activity is a cornerstone of weight management and overall health. In this section, we will explore the vital role exercise plays in achieving and maintaining a healthy weight, as well as provide simple and effective exercise routines that can easily fit into your daily life.

The Role of Exercise in Weight Management

1. Burning Calories: Exercise helps you burn calories, which is essential for weight loss and maintenance. When you engage in physical activities, your body uses energy, which can help create a calorie deficit needed for weight loss.

2. Building Muscle: Regular exercise, especially strength training, helps build muscle mass. Muscle burns more calories at rest than fat tissue, which means increasing your muscle mass can boost your metabolism and help you burn more calories throughout the day.

3. Reducing Fat: Exercise helps reduce body fat, including visceral fat, which is the dangerous fat that surrounds your internal organs and is linked to various health issues.

Exercise: Physical activity can enhance your metabolic rate both during exercise and after, through a process called excess post-exercise oxygen consumption (EPOC). This means your body continues to burn calories at a higher rate even after you've finished working out.

5. Enhancing Mood and Energy Levels: Regular physical activity boosts the release of endorphins, which are natural mood lifters. It can also improve your energy levels, making it easier to stay active and engaged in daily activities.

6.SupportingOverallHealth: Exercise helps reduce the risk of chronic diseases such as type 2 diabetes, heart disease, and certain cancers. It also strengthens your bones, improves cardiovascular health, and enhances flexibility and balance.

SIMPLE AND EFFECTIVE EXERCISE ROUTINE

Incorporating exercise into your daily routine doesn't have to be complicated or time-consuming. Here are some simple and effective exercises that can help you stay active and support your weight management goals:

1.CARDIOVASCULAR EXERCISES

Walking: Aim for at least 30 minutes of brisk walking most days of the week. Walking is an excellent low-impact exercise that can be done anywhere.

Running or Jogging: If you're up for a more intense workout, try running or jogging. Start with shorter distances and gradually increase your duration and intensity.

Cycling: Biking is a fun way to get your heart rate up. You can cycle outdoors or use a stationary bike at home or the gym.

Swimming: Swimming is a full-body workout that's easy on the joints. Try to swim for 30 minutes a few times a week.

2. STRENGTH TRAINING

Bodyweight Exercises: Incorporate exercises like push-ups, squats, lunges, and planks into your routine. These exercises don't require any equipment and can be done anywhere.

Resistance Bands: Resistance bands are portable and versatile. Use them for exercises like bicep curls, tricep extensions, and leg presses.

Weightlifting: If you have access to dumbbells or a gym, include weightlifting exercises such as deadlifts, bench presses, and shoulder presses to build muscle strength.

3. FLEXIBILITY AND BALANCE

Yoga: Practising yoga improves flexibility, strength, and balance. It's also great for stress relief and mindfulness.

Stretching: Incorporate stretching exercises into your daily routine to improve flexibility and prevent injuries. Focus on major muscle groups like your legs, back, and shoulders.

Tai Chi: This gentle form of exercise enhances balance and flexibility while also promoting relaxation.

4. HIGH-INTENSITY INTERVAL TRAINING (HIIT)

Short Bursts: HIIT involves alternating between short bursts of intense exercise and periods of rest or low-intensity exercise. This can be done with exercises like sprinting, jumping jacks, or burpees.

Efficiency: HIIT workouts are highly effective and can be completed in a shorter amount of time compared to traditional cardio workouts.

SAMPLE EXERCISE ROUTINE

Beginner Routine

Monday, Wednesday, Friday:

Warm-up: 5 minutes of light cardio (e.g., walking or jogging in place)

Bodyweight exercises: 3 sets of 10-15 reps each (squats, push-ups, lunges)

Cardio: 20 minutes of brisk walking or cycling

Cool-down: 10 minutes of stretching

Intermediate Routine

Tuesday, Thursday, Saturday:

Warm-up: 5 minutes of light cardio

HIIT: 20 minutes (30 seconds of sprinting, 1 minute of walking)

Strength training: 3 sets of 10-15 reps each (dumbbell curls, shoulder presses, deadlifts)

Cool-down: 5 minutes of stretching

Advanced Routine
Monday to Saturday:

Warm-up: 5-15 minutes of light cardio

Mixed workout: 30 minutes (combining cardio, strength, and flexibility exercises)

Cool-down: 5-15 minutes of stretching or yoga

Regular exercise, combined with a healthy diet, is a powerful combination for achieving and maintaining a healthy weight. Start with the routines that match your fitness level and gradually increase the intensity as you become more comfortable. Stay consistent, and you'll soon see the benefits of a more active lifestyle.

MINDSET AND MOTIVATION

Overcoming Challenges and Setbacks

Every journey has its ups and downs, and this weight loss journey is no different. It's important to recognize that challenges and setbacks are a natural part of the process. What matters most is how you see them.

1. Acknowledge Setbacks:

Understand that setbacks are normal and can happen to anyone. Whether it's a missed workout, an indulgent meal, or a temporary lapse in motivation, acknowledge it without judgement. Remember, one setback doesn't define your entire journey.

2. Learn from Mistakes: Each setback is an opportunity to learn. Reflect on what triggered it and how you can avoid similar situations in the future. For instance, if stress led to emotional eating, consider developing healthier coping mechanisms like exercise, meditation, or talking to a friend.

3. Plan Ahead: Anticipate potential challenges and plan accordingly. If you know you have a busy week ahead, prepare healthy meals in advance or schedule shorter, more intense workouts that fit into your schedule. Having a plan can help you stay on track even when life gets hectic.

4. Stay Flexible: Life is unpredictable, and sometimes things don't go as planned. Be flexible and adapt to changes. If you can't stick to your routine, find alternative ways to stay active and make healthier food choices. A 10-minute walk is better than no walk at all.

5. Celebrate Small Wins: Acknowledge and celebrate your progress, no matter how small. Did you choose a healthy snack instead of junk food? Did you complete a workout even when you didn't feel like it? Celebrating these small victories can boost your motivation and remind you of how far you've come.

Developing a Positive Mindset for Long-Term Success

A positive mindset is crucial for achieving long-term success in your weight loss journey. It's about cultivating a mental attitude that supports your goals and helps you stay committed, even when the going gets tough.

1. Set Realistic Goals: Establish achievable, realistic goals that keep you motivated and focused. Break your larger goals into smaller, manageable steps. For example, instead of aiming to lose 20 pounds, start with a goal of losing 5 pounds and build from there.

2. Practice Self-Compassion: Be kind to yourself. Avoid negative self-talk and treat yourself with the same compassion you would offer a friend. Understand that progress takes time, and it's okay to make mistakes along the way.

3. Visualise Success: Spend a few minutes each day visualising your success. Imagine how you will feel, look, and what you will be able to do once you reach your goals. This can help reinforce your commitment and keep you motivated.

4. Staying Positive: Surround yourself with positive influences, whether it's supportive friends and family or motivational quotes and books. Positivity can be contagious and can help you maintain a hopeful and determined outlook.

5. Focusing on Health, Not Just Weight: Shift your focus from purely losing weight to improving your overall health and well-being. Celebrate non-scale victories such as increased energy levels, improved mood, and better sleep. These are equally important indicators of your progress.

6. Keep Learning: Stay informed about healthy living by reading books, attending workshops, or joining support groups. Knowledge empowers you to make better choices and stay motivated.

7. Building Support System: Surround yourself with people who support your goals and encourage you. Share your journey with them and don't hesitate to ask for help when you need it. Having a strong support system can make a significant difference in your success.

Adopting a positive mindset and staying motivated are key components of your weight loss journey. By overcoming challenges and developing mental resilience, you're setting yourself up for long-term success. Remember, it's not just about the destination, but also about enjoying and learning from the journey. Keep going, stay positive, and believe in yourself you've got this.

REAL LIFE SUCCESS STORIES

Inspirational Journeys from Others Who Have Succeeded

Reading about the successes of others can be incredibly motivating. Here are a few real-life success stories from individuals who have embarked on their own 21-day dieting journeys and achieved remarkable results. Let these stories inspire you and remind you that you, too, can succeed.

1. Esther 's Journey: From Fast Food to Fresh Food

Esther, a 35-year-old teacher, struggled with obesity for years. Her busy schedule led her to rely heavily on fast food, and she rarely found time for exercise. When her doctor warned her about the health risks associated with her weight, she knew it was time for a change.

Challenge: Esther found it difficult to break her fast food habit and incorporate healthy meals into her routine.

Approach: She started by meal prepping on Sundays, making healthy lunches and dinners that she could quickly reheat during the week. She also began taking a 30 minute walk every evening.

Success: Over the course of the 21-day plan, Esther lost 10 pounds and reported feeling more energetic and focused. Her new habits have become a sustainable part of her lifestyle, and she continues to see progress.

2. Mike's Transformation: From Couch Potato to Fitness Enthusiast

Mike, a 28-year-old software engineer, led a sedentary lifestyle, spending most of his day sitting at a desk and his evenings on the couch. At his annual check-up, he was shocked to learn he was prediabetic and needed to make immediate changes.

Challenge: Mike needed to find a way to integrate physical activity into his daily routine and improve his diet.

Approach: He started with simple changes, like swapping sugary drinks for water and adding short workouts during his lunch break. He followed the 21-day meal plan, focusing on balanced, nutritious meals.

Success: By the end of the 21 days, Mike had lost 12 pounds and reduced his blood sugar levels significantly. He discovered a love for running and has since completed his first 5K race.

3. Sophia's Story: Overcoming Emotional Eating

Sophia, a 40-year-old mother of two, struggled with emotional eating, especially during stressful times. This led to a gradual weight gain that she found hard to reverse.

Challenge: Sophia needed to address her emotional eating habits and find healthier ways to cope with stress.

Approach: She began practising mindfulness and keeping a food diary to track her eating patterns. Sophia also started attending a weekly yoga class to help manage stress.

Success: In 21 days, Sophia lost 8 pounds and gained a greater understanding of her emotional triggers. She continues to practise mindfulness and yoga, which have helped her maintain her weight and improve her overall well-being.

4. John's Success: The Power of Community Support

John, a 50-year-old construction worker, had always been overweight but found it especially challenging to lose weight as he got older. He decided to join a local weight loss group for support and accountability.

Challenge: John needed consistent motivation and support to stick to his weight loss plan.

Approach: He followed the 21-day diet plan and regularly attended group meetings where he shared his progress and challenges. The community support kept him accountable and motivated.

Success: John lost 15 pounds in 21 days and found a new sense of community. The encouragement from his group helped him stay committed, and he continues to attend meetings and inspire others with his journey.

These real-life success stories illustrate that with determination, support, and the right strategies, achieving your weight loss goals is possible. Whether you're overcoming emotional eating, breaking unhealthy habits, or finding new ways to stay active, remember that every small step brings you closer to your goal. Let these stories be a testament to the power of commitment and the positive changes that are within your reach.

ADDITIONAL RESOURCES

1. The Obesity Code by Dr. Jason Fung

Dr. Fung explores the underlying causes of obesity and offers practical advice on how to address them. This book is a great resource for understanding the science behind weight gain and effective strategies for weight loss.

2. The Whole30: The 30-Day Guide to Total Health and Food Freedom by Melissa Hartwig Urban and Dallas Hartwig

This guide provides a structured plan for eliminating unhealthy foods and resetting your body. It's an excellent resource for those looking to make a significant lifestyle change.

3. Intuitive Eating: A Revolutionary Program That Works by Evelyn Tribole and Elyse Resch

Learn how to develop a healthier relationship with food, reject diet culture, and trust your body's natural hunger cues. This book is perfect for those who struggle with emotional eating.

4. Atomic Habits: An Easy & Proven Way to Build Good Habits & Break Bad Ones by James Clear.
 Clear's book on habit formation is invaluable for anyone looking to make lasting changes. It offers practical tips for developing healthy habits that stick.

5. The Mayo Clinic Diet: Eat Well. Enjoy Life. Lose Weight. by the Mayo Clinic
 A comprehensive guide to losing weight in a healthy and sustainable way, this book provides practical advice, meal plans, and recipes to support your journey.

Online Communities and Support Groups

1. MyFitnessPal Community

An active community of people who share tips, recipes, and support each other's fitness journeys. It's a great place to find motivation and accountability.

2. Reddit: lose it

This subreddit is dedicated to weight loss support and provides a platform for sharing success stories, asking for advice, and getting encouragement from others on a similar path.

3. SparkPeople

A free online community with resources, articles, and forums where you can connect with others, track your progress, and find support.

4. Weight Watchers Connect

For those following the Weight Watchers program, Connect is a supportive social network where members share their journeys, tips, and encouragement.

5. Facebook Groups

Search for groups focused on weight loss, healthy eating, or specific diet plans. These groups can offer a sense of community and support, with members sharing their experiences and advice.

Useful Tools and Apps for Diet and Exercise Tracking

1. MyFitnessPal

This app allows you to track your food intake, exercise, and weight. It has a vast database of foods and a barcode scanner to make logging meals easy.

2. Lose It

Similar to MyFitnessPal, Lose It! helps you set weight loss goals, track your food intake, and monitor your progress. It also includes a barcode scanner and community features.

3. Fitbit

Track your daily activity, workouts, and sleep patterns with a Fitbit device. The accompanying app provides detailed insights and allows you to set fitness goals.

4. Cronometer

This app offers detailed nutrient tracking, helping you ensure you're getting the right balance of vitamins and minerals. It's especially useful for those with specific dietary needs.

5. Nike Training Club

Access a variety of workouts ranging from yoga to high-intensity interval training (HIIT). The app offers guided sessions that can be done at home or the gym.

6. Headspace

Incorporate mindfulness and stress management into your routine with this meditation app. It offers guided meditations to help you stay calm and focused.

The additional resources are designed to support your journey towards better health and weight management. From insightful books and supportive online communities to practical tools and apps, you have everything you need to stay informed, motivated, and on track. Remember, we are in this journey together, leverage these resources to build a strong support system to achieve your goals.

CONCLUSION

Celebrating Progress

Reflect on the journey you've taken towards achieving your goals. Celebrate the milestones both big and small. Acknowledge the effort and dedication you made to get to this point. Whether improving health, learning new skills, or making positive lifestyle changes, take time to appreciate how far you've come.

Maintaining Your New Lifestyle

Set Sustainment Goals: Define how you will maintain the progress you've made. Establish specific, realistic goals that align with your new lifestyle. This could include daily habits, weekly routines, or long term commitments.

Create a Support System: Identify people or resources that can help you stay accountable and motivated. This might involve joining a community of like-minded individuals, finding a mentor, or regularly checking in with a supportive friend or family member.

Adaptability and Flexibility: Understand that maintaining a new lifestyle involves adapting to challenges and changes. Stay flexible in your approach and be willing to adjust your goals when needed.

Celebrate Consistently: Incorporate regular celebrations of your achievements into your maintenance plan. This can help reinforce positive behaviors and provide motivation to continue.

Reflect and Learn: Periodically review your progress and reflect on what has worked well and what could be improved. Use this self-reflection to refine your maintenance strategy and set new goals for continued.

Caloric Intake: The number of calories consumed through food and drink.

BMI (Body Mass Index): A measurement that assesses body weight relative to height.

Macronutrients: Nutrients needed in large amounts, including carbohydrates, proteins, and fats.

Micronutrients: Essential vitamins and minerals required in smaller quantities for health.

Metabolism: The process by which the body converts food into energy.

Saturated Fat: A type of fat found in animal products and some plant oils, which can raise cholesterol levels.

Trans Fat: An unhealthy fat often found in processed foods, which can increase the risk of heart disease.

This appendix provides practical resources such as measurement conversion charts and a glossary of terms related to health, nutrition, and weight management, enhancing the usability and educational value of your document.

Bonus
7-Day Healthy Habit Booster Plan

Kickstart your ongoing journey to health with our complimentary 7-day Healthy Habit Booster Plan. This supplementary guide is designed to reinforce and build on the habits you've established during your 21-day journey with 21-Day Dieting for Obesity.

DAY 1: Morning Routine
Start your day with a glass of lemon water to hydrate and detoxify your body.

Practice 15 minutes of mindfulness or gentle stretching exercises.

DAY 2: Balanced Meals
-Plan and prepare a balanced breakfast, lunch, and dinner using the recipes from the book.
- Include a variety of colourful fruits and vegetables in each meal.

DAY 3: Physical Activity
Engage in 35 minutes of moderate intensity exercise, such as brisk walking or swimming.

Incorporate strength training exercises to build lean muscle mass.

DAY 4: Mindful Eating
Practise mindful eating techniques, such as chewing slowly and savouring each bite.
 Avoid distractions like screens or reading while eating.

DAY 5: Hydration
 Aim to drink at least 8 glasses of water throughout the day.
 Include herbal teas or infused water for added flavour and hydration.

DAY 6: Healthy Snacking
 Prepare nutritious snacks like fresh fruit, yoghourt with nuts, or vegetable sticks with hummus.
 Avoid sugary or processed snacks.

DAY 7: Reflection and Planning
 Reflect on your progress over the past week and celebrate your achievements.
Plan your meals and physical activity for the upcoming week to stay on track with your goals.

This 7-day Healthy Habit Booster Plan complements 21-Day Dieting for Obesity, by providing practical steps and daily activities to support long term success in maintaining a healthy lifestyle. Use this guide to continue building healthy habits and achieving your wellness goals.

<u>Thank You</u>

Dear Reader,

Thank you so much for purchasing 21-Day Dieting for Obesity. Your support means the world to me, and I am truly grateful that you chose this book to help guide you on your journey to a healthier life.

Wrote this book with you in mind, hoping to provide a practical and effective plan to help you achieve your weight loss goals. I understand that dealing with obesity can be challenging, but I believe that with the right tools and information in this book, you can take control of your health and make lasting positive changes.

Your decision to buy this book shows that you are committed to making a difference in your life. I hope you find the 21-day meal plan, recipes, and practical tips helpful and motivating. Each small step you take brings you closer to a healthier, happier you.

I would love to hear about your experience with the book. Your feedback is incredibly valuable to me and helps me improve and create more useful content. If you enjoyed the book and found it helpful, please consider leaving a review on Amazon. Your reviews help others find this book and start their own journey to better health.

Thank you once again for your support. I wish you all the best on your journey to managing your weight and living a healthier, happier life.

With gratitude,
Aurora Grace.

www.ingramcontent.com/pod-product-compliance
Lightning Source LLC
Chambersburg PA
CBHW051705250726
48653CB00007B/2871